Keto Diet After 50

The Complete Guide to Ketogenic Diet for Men and Women Over 50...Includes Quick and Easy Recipes for Losing Weight and Many Meal Plans

1

Table of Contents

Table of Contents

Introduction

Congratulations on buying *Keto Diet After 50.* Thanks a lot for doing so.
There are various types of diet plans that can be found today for losing weight. But, there are only a few diet plans that are effective even after the age of 50. The ketogenic diet falls under this group. This diet plan is based on low carb consumption. If you are above the age of 50 and willing to start with a proper diet plan, this book has all the information you need. The keto diet is very effective in losing weight, besides keeping you healthy and fit. When you get the opportunity to start with a proper diet plan that perfectly suits your age group, building your long-desired body will become easier, and so will its maintenance. If you are not familiar with a low carb diet, starting with the keto diet might sound a bit tough. However, with time as you get the desired results, it will become easier for you.
The keto diet meal plans are often treated as being controversial. The primary reason behind this is most people think the high-fat content of the meals can increase the body's cholesterol level. However, according to some recent studies, following a diet low on carbs has its own benefits. The recipes you will come across in this book can help start with the keto diet very easily .
You can find lots of books based on this subject in today's market. Thank you again for selecting this one! Every effort was given to make sure this book is filled with as much beneficial information as possible. So, please enjoy it!

Chapter 1: How to Begin With a Keto Diet After 50

The ketogenic diet is a long-known diet plan that is very effective in losing extra weight. It is low in carbs and is high in fat consumption. It has been found that the keto diet is can in improving the quality of your health besides shedding extra weight. It can impart several other types of benefits on the body against epilepsy, diabetes, cancer, and Alzheimer's disease. Several studies found that the keto diet is more popular among women as it can show positive results in dealing with the various symptoms of menopause. Some of the most common menopause symptoms are irritability, fatigue, and sudden increase in body weight. Various researches claim that the keto diet can very easily deal with all these symptoms. But is it really so? Are you thinking of starting with the diet but not sure where to start from? This section has got all that you need.

Basics About the Keto Diet

The keto diet or ketogenic diet is a low-carb diet. It has several similarities with the low-carb and Atkins diet. The main aim of this diet is to reduce your intake of carbohydrates drastically. You will need to replace the same with healthy fats. As you reduce the consumption of carbohydrates drastically, the body will enter a metabolic state. This state is known as ketosis. When ketosis occurs, your body will become more efficient in burning out all the fat to provide energy to the body for carrying out various basic functions. It will also turn the body fats into ketones in your liver that helps supply the required energy to the brain. The keto diet also reduces the levels of insulin and blood sugar drastically. This, in addition to the increased number of ketones, comes with several other health benefits.

Ketogenic Diet for Losing Weight

The keto diet is a very effective and easy way of losing extra pounds from your body. It also helps to cut off the risk factors of various diseases. It has been found that this diet is even more effective than various other low-fat diets. Additionally, the keto diet is so filling in nature that you will be able to shed all the extra weight without counting on calories or keeping track of food consumption. In a study, it has been stated that people who follow the keto diet can lose about two times more weight in comparison to those people who are on a calorie-restricted and low-fat diet. The HDL cholesterol level, along with the levels of triglyceride, also gets improved.

Ketogenic Diet for Prediabetes and Diabetes

Diabetes is most often characterized by various metabolic state changes, impaired functioning of insulin, and high blood sugar levels. The keto diet can reduce excess fat, which can be linked to metabolic syndrome, type 2 diabetes, and prediabetes. According to the latest study, this diet plan can improve sensitivity to insulin by almost 75%. So, it can be said that this diet can easily help in dealing with diabetes, along with its various characteristics.

Several Other Health Benefits Related to the Keto Diet

There are various other benefits of the keto diet besides weight loss and dealing with diabetes.

Cancer: This diet plan is now being adapted to treat various cancer types and slow tumor growth.

Alzheimer's disease: According to recent studies, the keto diet can help in dealing with Alzheimer's disease and slow its progression speed.

Polycystic ovary syndrome: The keto diet effectively reduces insulin levels, which can play an important role in reducing polycystic ovary syndrome.

Increase in the level of HDL cholesterol: HDL cholesterol is known as good cholesterol. The keto diet can increase HDL levels by lowering the intake of carbohydrates and consuming more fats. This will help to lower the risks of various heart-related diseases or even heart attacks.

Better sleep: It has been found that even a small quantity of glucose in the diet is very effective in disturbing the blood sugar levels in the body. It will ultimately lead to poor or bad sleep. As you grow with age, the quality of sleep is most likely to degrade. When you start following the keto diet, it can help keep blood sugar levels under proper control. Additionally, it can also help balance the levels of other types of hormones like cortisol and melatonin.

How Can You Easily Start the Diet?

Adapting the keto diet is not at all tough. However, you will need to take care of certain things for the best possible results.

Having a clear idea of what foods to consume and what to avoid: It is very important to understand what food items you can consume and whatnot. You will need to concentrate on limiting the intake of carbs with more focus on healthy fats.

Examine your connection with healthy fats: For starting with a diet high in fats, you will need to start with very small adjustments. It might turn out to be uncomfortable at the beginning. But, making small changes every day can help in easing the process for you.

Plan a starting date: A very important thing that you will need to ensure is to sort out your entire diet schedule. Start by fixing a date and start from that day only. In case you have any parties or other plans with your friends, try to share your target with them. It will help you to get all the support you need for starting with the diet plan.

Limiting the daily carbohydrate intake to 20 grams: As you start to push your body towards ketosis, it is very important for you that you start consuming lots of healthy fats. As the ketogenic diet's primary motive is to lower the intake of carbohydrates, make sure that your daily intake of carbs does not go beyond 20 grams. It is a very important step. What you can do is that you can add more fat along with proteins for filling up that space. Maintaining the ratio of carbs to fat is very important for supplying the body with the required amount of ketones.

Chapter 2: Why Is It Hard to Lose Weight After 50 and Effects of Aging on Nutritional Needs

All those diets that worked out so well during your 20s, 30s, or 40s do not seem to work like before after crossing the mark of 50. Why so? Are you not hitting your treadmill hard or consuming too many carbs? Losing weight after the age of 50 and beyond is a completely different game. You might think that it is very hard or impossible to shed those extra pounds after 50. But, you still have the opportunity to eliminate those extra pounds. All you need to do is determine all those hurdles that are standing in front of you.

You Are Experiencing Muscle Loss Due to Age

The total amount of lean muscle that you have naturally will start to decline by 4 to 7 percent every decade after crossing the mark of 30. This process is known as sarcopenia. You might also start losing muscles if you are not that active because of various health conditions related to age, such as arthritis. Getting a surgery or injury after 30 can also lead to the same. All of these instances might not lead to any significant kind of decline. However, cumulatively, they all do. Why does muscle loss matter? The main logic behind this is that the lean muscles tend to use up more calories than fat. So, if you are not training your strength daily with weights for building and maintaining muscle, there will be fewer needs of calories every day. It can lead to weight gain if you keep consuming the same number of calories exactly like when you were younger.

Majority of the people have the tendency not to adjust their calorie consumption as they age. They will just keep on eating the same. As they possess lean muscle mass for burning all those calories and less percentage of activity, the result is weight gain.

Normal Changes in Hormone Levels

Every human being undergoes several changes in their levels of hormones as a normal part of their aging. It can easily explain why mid-age is the pick time of putting on extra pounds. For women, the onset of menopause, which typically occurs between the age of forty-five and fifty-five, results in a drastic drop in estrogen levels. This tends to encourage the accumulation of extra pounds near the belly very easily. This kind of shift in the storage of fats can make the gain of weight even more noticeable. It can also make a sudden rise in the overall risk of high blood pressure, heart disease, diabetes, and high cholesterol. Also, fluctuations in estrogen levels during perimenopause, the years before menopause, can result in mood swings. This kind of sudden mood swings might make it tougher to just stick to an exercise plan along with a healthy diet .

For men, there is a sudden change in the levels of testosterone with age. The testosterone level tends to decline gradually around the age of 40 by two to three percent every year. Besides other things, testosterone is responsible for regulating fat distribution along with muscle mass and strength. In simple terms, reduction in testosterone levels can result in making the body less effective in burning calories.

With age, the growth hormone which is produced by the pituitary gland also reduces in percentage. One of the primary functions of the growth hormone is to maintain and build muscle mass. So, when the level of growth hormone decreases, it gets tougher for the body to build and maintain the mass of muscles.

The Rate of Metabolism Becomes Slow

When there is a decrease in muscle mass, the body's metabolic rate tends to slow down. Metabolism is a very complex process that helps in the conversion of calories into useful energy. Having less muscle and more fat will reduce the calorie-burning process. Also, many people tend to get less active with growing age. It can also slow down the metabolism. Age is not the primary thing that can determine the metabolic rate. The sex and size of the body also play important roles. Certain types of health conditions, like hypothyroidism, can also affect the rate of metabolism .

More Stress and Less Activity

As you reach the age of fifty, your work schedule or career is most likely to be in full swing. This can lead to certain challenges in weight loss. You will be moving less, commute to your work by seating for an hour and work at the desk for seven or more hours. You will already have so much served on the plate that you will find it difficult to take out some time for exercise or a short walk during the day. With more work pressure, you will get more stress as well. It can result in a sudden boost in ghrelin levels, the hormone that can make you hungrier. You will end up consuming more calories. Ultimately this will lead to weight increase.

Not Enough Sleep

Not getting enough sleep and sleep disturbances are very common as you cross the mark of 50. For women, menopause can lead to sleep disruptions because of hot flashes or even arthritis. When you do not get enough sleep, it readily affects the overall production of the growth hormone. Growth hormone is essential for muscle and bone mass.

Relation Between Aging and Nutritional Needs

While talking about aging, it can be related to several types of body changes, for instance, muscle loss, thinner skin, less stomach acid, and many others. Most of these can lead to nutrient deficiency, while others might directly affect the quality of life and the senses. For instance, it has been found that approximately 27% of elderly people tend to suffer from atrophic gastritis. It is a condition that leads to the chronic nature of inflammation along with cellular damage. All of these are responsible for the production of stomach acid. As the level of acid in our stomach gets low, it can readily affect the absorption of nutrients like vitamin B12, iron, calcium, and magnesium.

Malnutrition can be treated as both a consequence and a cause of ill health. It might be of several types, such as overnutrition, undernutrition, or even specific nutrition deficiencies. Malnutrition in aging people, is most of the time, underdiagnosed. Malnutrition in people who have crossed the 50 mark can result in various health problems and a weaker immune system. When you tend to have a weak immune system, there is most likely to be an increase in the risk of infections, muscle weakness, and poor healing of wounds.

Including More Fiber in Daily Diet

Constipation is among the most common problems that can be found in elderly people. Constipation is more common among all those people who are above the age of 50.

According to some studies, women tend to suffer more from constipation as compared to men. The development of constipation, along with growing age, comes along with a definite reason. As with growing age, you are most likely to have lesser movements. You might also need to consume various types of medications. In such cases, constipation might develop as a definite side effect. But, how to get rid of this? The solution is simple. You will need to consume more fiber. Fiber can very easily pass through the gut even in its undigested form. So, it can help in the proper passing of stool with even movements of the bowel. Also, as you start consuming more fiber, it can help in the prevention of diverticular disease. It is a serious condition in which various small structures develop along the colon wall.

Need for More Nutrients and Fewer Calories

The daily amount of calories needed by a person relies on several factors like weight, activity level, muscle mass, height, and various others. Elderly adults and people above the age of 50 require fewer calories. The primary reason behind this is less amount of exercise and lesser movements. When you continue consuming the same number of calories per day, just like the days when you were younger, it will result in fat gain. The fat gain can be seen mainly near the belly area. Although the need for calories is much less, there is a high need for various other types of nutrients. That is why people above the age of 50 need to consume several types of whole food items such as lean meat, fish, and veggies. Whole food can help in dealing with a deficiency of nutrients without any effect on the waistline. Some examples of essential nutrients are vitamin B12, vitamin D, calcium, protein, and others.

Increased Need for Vitamin B12

Vitamin B12 belongs to the group of essential nutrients that are required with growing age. The most important function carried out by this vitamin is the production of red blood cells. Not only that, but vitamin B12 is also responsible for proper brain functioning. According to some recent studies, about 25-30% of people who have crossed the 50 mark are most likely to have reduced ability to absorb vitamin B12 from the diet they follow. So, with passing time, it can eventually lead to vitamin B12 deficiency. Vitamin B12 comes along with all those proteins that we consume daily. Before the body can use up this vitamin, the stomach acids help separate the same from the proteins. With growing age, the production of acid in the stomach is most likely to decrease. So, this might result in lesser absorption of this important vitamin from our daily diet.

Importance of Calcium and Vitamin D

We all know that vitamin D, along with calcium, is essential for maintaining the bones' proper health. Calcium is responsible for building up and maintenance of healthy bones. On the other hand, vitamin D helps in the absorption of calcium by the body. However, elderly people can absorb less amount of calcium from their daily diet. It has been found that the gut tends to absorb less calcium with growing age. But, the primary reason behind the decrease in calcium absorption is vitamin D deficiency. Vitamin D can be produced by the human body from the available cholesterol in the skin when exposed to the sunlight. As we grow old, our skin also becomes thinner. So, the ability of the skin to produce vitamin D also gets reduced.

So, because of vitamin D and calcium deficiency, our bone health will also decrease. Thus, the risk of fractures and injuries will tend to increase. Green leafy vegetables, along with dairy products, are great sources of calcium. Vitamin D is available in several types of fish like salmon, herring, and others.
There are several other types of nutrients that you will need with growing age. Some of them are:

Magnesium: This nutrient aids in the process of digestion as it tends to get disrupted with age. It is very important besides vitamin and calcium.

Potassium: As you increase the consumption of potassium, the risks of osteoporosis, kidney stones, heart diseases, and high blood pressure will also get reduced.

Iron: Deficiency of iron can lead to anemia, which is very common in elderly people. It is a condition where oxygen is deficient in the blood.

Omega-3 fatty acid: It is very important for heart health. It can also help in lowering high blood pressure.

With growing age, maintaining a proper proportion of nutrients is very important. The diet that you will choose will determine the kind of life that you will have.

Chapter 3: Keto Diet Food List

The ketogenic diet is all about restricting the consumption of carbohydrates. Typically, carbs are regarded as the preferred energy source of the body. However, when you are on a strict keto diet, the energy intake from carbs will be even less than five percent. That is what triggers the process of ketosis in the body. Even when you have a clear idea that you will need to concentrate on eating high-fat low-carb food items, it might still turn out to be a bit confusing as to which food items you can eat. In this chapter, you will find most of the food items you can consume while on a ketogenic diet.

Seafood and Fish

Fish is a great source of selenium, B vitamins, and potassium. Additionally, it is rich in proteins and is free from carbs as well. Sardines, salmons, albacore tuna, mackerel, and other fatty fish types come with a great percentage of omega-3 fatty acids. If you want to lower your blood sugar levels, omega-3 fatty acids can help you a lot. It can also increase the sensitivity to insulin. Frequent fish consumption can be linked with a decreased risk of various types of chronic diseases and great mental health.

Low-Carb Vegetable s

Non-starchy vegetables are low in carbs as well as calories. They are rich in various types of nutrients, like vitamin C and essential minerals. Low-carb veggies are rich in antioxidants that can help in protecting against the free radicals that damage cells. You can aim to consume non-starchy veggies with about eight grams of net carbs for each cup. Some great options for low-carb veggies are cauliflower, broccoli, bell peppers, green beans, spinach, and zucchini. You can very easily substitute high-carb foods with vegetables. For instance, cauliflower can be used in place of rice or mashed potatoes, or you can also substitute noodles with zoodles made from zucchini and many others.

Cheese

Cheese falls under the group of food items that are tasty and rich in nutrients as well. There are various cheese types that can be found in the market. Fortunately, cheeses of all types are high in fat and are low in carbs. So, you can consider cheese as a perfect food item that can be included in your ketogenic diet plan. Consuming one ounce of cheese can provide your body with seven grams of protein, one gram of carbs, and fifteen percent RDI for calcium. Majority of the people think of cheese as being unhealthy as it is rich in saturated fat. However, cheese consumption has still not shown any sign in increasing the overall risk of heart diseases. Additionally, cheese also comes with linoleic acid, which is most often related to fat loss. Cheese is a great food item that can help in muscle mass retention, which generally reduces with growing age.

Avocado

Avocado can be included in your ketogenic diet plan as a heart-healthy fat. It is rich in potassium and fat. Consuming half an avocado will provide you with only nine grams of carbs, out of which seven grams are fiber. Shifting to plant fats from animal fats can help in readily improving the levels of triglyceride and cholesterol.

Eggs

Eggs are a great source of minerals, proteins, B vitamins, and antioxidants. Consuming two eggs every day will provide you with zero carbs and twelve grams of protein. Eggs can trigger hormones that can help to increase the feeling of fullness. It can also help in stabilizing the levels of blood sugar. Eggs come with antioxidants such as zeaxanthin and lutein, which can help maintain the eyes' proper health. Also, many people only consume the white portion of the egg. However, the majority of the nutrients are present in the egg yolk. So, it is essential to consume a complete egg.

Meat and Poultry

Meat is an important source of lean proteins and is also considered a staple on the keto diet. Fresh poultry and meat come with zero carbs and are also rich in B vitamins and various types of minerals, such as selenium, potassium, and zinc. Although processed meats, such as sausage and bacon, are permitted in the keto diet, they are not good for your heart's health. Excessive consumption of processed meats can also increase the overall risk of developing cancer. Try to limit processed meat as much as possible and opt for fresh meat and poultry.

Healthy Oils, Seeds, and Nuts

Seeds and nuts are rich in monounsaturated and polyunsaturated fats, protein, and fiber. They are also excessively low in net carb count. Coconut oil, along with olive oil, are the two recommended types of oils while being on a keto diet. Olive oil is rich in oleic acid. It can also be linked to lower risks of heart diseases. Coconut oil is a great source of saturated fats but also comes with MCTs or medium-chain triglycerides. It can readily help in increasing the overall production of ketones. MCTs can also help in improving the rate of metabolism and can promote weight loss and reduction of belly fat as well.

Unsweetened Tea and Coffee

Plain tea and coffee come with zero carbohydrates. So, they can be regarded as a perfect fit for the keto diet. It has been found that coffee can lower the overall risk of cardiovascular disease and type 2 diabetes. Tea comes with less caffeine and is high in antioxidants in comparison to coffee. It can help in weight loss, boost your immune system's functioning, and reduce stroke and heart attack risk.

Berries

Berries are a great source of antioxidants. They can help in protecting against diseases and can also reduce inflammation. They come with high fiber content and are low in carbs. Net carb count for half a cup of some common berries:

Raspberries: Nine grams of net carbs
Blackberries: Three grams of net carbs
Strawberries: Three grams of net carbs
Blueberries: Nine grams of net carbs

Chapter 4: Three-Week Keto Meal Plan

In this chapter, you will find a keto meal plan for twenty-one days, where your only aim will be to maintain the calorie count each day. The recipes are flexible, and you can replace any of the ingredients with ingredients of your choice to fit your liking. You can alter the recipes in this twenty-one days meal plan. Let us start with the breakfast plan first.

Breakfast Keto Meal Plan

Breakfast is most often regarded as an essential meal in a day. In this section, you will come across various breakfast recipes that can be altered in the twenty-one days meal challenge. Majority of the nutritionists suggest opting for a fulfilling breakfast so that you can stay full majority of the day.

Keto Fresh Spinach Frittata

Total Prep & Cooking Time: Forty-five minutes
Yields: Four servings
Nutrition Facts: Calories: 462.3 | Protein: 28.3g | Carbs: 3.4g| Fat: 47.6g | Fiber: 1.3g

Ingredients

- Five ounces of diced chorizo or bacon
- Two tbsps. of butter
- Eight ounces of spinach (fresh, chopped)
- Eight large eggs
- One cup of heavy cream (whipped)
- Five ounces of cheese (shredded)
- Pepper and salt (for seasoning)

Method:

1. Preheat your oven at one-hundred and seventy-five degrees Celsius. Grease a large baking dish with the help of cooking spray.
2. Heat the butter in an iron skillet. Add the chorizo. Fry until crispy. Add the chopped spinach. Cook for three minutes until wilted. Remove the skillet from the heat. Keep aside.
3. Whisk the cream along with the eggs in a large mixing bowl. Pour the egg mixture into the greased baking dish.
4. Add the spinach and bacon mix from the top. Add the cheese.
5. Bake for thirty minutes.

Baked Bacon Omelet

Total Prep & Cooking Time: Twenty-five minutes
Yields: Two servings
Nutrition Facts: Calories: 623.6 | Protein: 22.6g | Carbs: 2g| Fat: 71.3g | Fiber: 1.6g

Ingredients

- Four large eggs
- Five ounces of bacon (cubed)
- Three ounces of butter
- Two ounces of spinach (fresh)

One tbsp. of chives (chopped)
Pepper and salt (for seasoning)

Method:

1. Preheat your oven at two hundred degrees Celsius. Use butter for greasing a baking dish.
2. Heat remaining butter in an iron skillet. Fry the bacon cubes for one minute. Add the spinach and mix well.
3. Whisk the eggs in a medium-sized bowl. Combine the bacon spinach mixture. Mix properly.
4. Add pepper and salt. Add the chives and stir.
5. Pour the prepared mixture of egg into the greased baking dish.
6. Bake for twenty minutes.
7. Serve hot.

Keto Pancake With Whipped Cream and Berries

Total Prep & Cooking Time: Twenty-five minutes

Yields: Four servings

Nutrition Facts: Calories: 421.6 | Protein: 14.6g | Carbs: 3.4g| Fat: 41.3g | Fiber: 3.2g

Ingredients

For the pancakes:

- Four large eggs
- Seven ounces of cottage cheese
- One tbsp. of ground psyllium husk powder
- Two ounces of butter

For the toppings:

- Two ounces of raspberries
- One cup of whipping cream

Method:

1. Combine together cottage cheese, eggs, and husk powder in a bowl. Mix well. Let the mixture sit for ten minutes.
2. Heat the butter in an iron skillet. Add half cup of the pancake mixture. Fry for four minutes on each side. Repeat with the remaining batter.
3. Add the whipping cream to a bowl. Keep whipping until it forms soft peaks.
4. Serve the pancakes in serving plates. Top with whipped cream and raspberries.

Coconut Porridge

Total Prep & Cooking Time: Ten minutes
Yields: Two servings
Nutrition Facts: Calories: 436.3 | Protein: 10.2g | Carbs: 3.2g| Fat: 49.3g | Fiber: 5.2g

Ingredients

- One large egg (beaten)
- One tbsp. of coconut flour
- One pinch of ground psyllium husk powder
- Half tsp. of salt
- One ounce of butter
- Four tbsps. of coconut cream

Method:

1. Combine husk powder, coconut flour, salt, and egg in a medium-sized bowl.
2. Take a small pan. Heat the butter. Add the coconut cream and mix. Whisk in the mixture of egg slowly. Keep combining until the texture is thick and creamy.
3. Serve immediately with coconut cream.

Western Omelet

Total Prep & Cooking Time: Thirty minutes
Yields: Two servings
Nutrition Facts: Calories: 623.1 | Protein: 41.6g | Carbs: 6.3g| Fat: 57.6g | Fiber: 1.1g

Ingredients

Six large eggs
Two tbsps. of sour cream
Pepper and salt (for seasoning)
Three ounces of cheese (shredded)
Two ounces of butter
Five ounces of smoked deli ham (diced)
Half yellow onion (chopped)
Half green bell pepper (chopped)

Method:

1. Whisk the cream along with the eggs in a bowl. Keep whisking until fluffy.
2. Add half of the cheese. Mix well.
3. Melt the butter in a large pan. Add the ham. SauteL for one minute. Add the onion along with the green bell pepper. SauteL for one minute.
4. Add the mixture of eggs. Keep cooking until the egg is set.
5. Lower the flame. Add remaining cheese from the top. Fold the omelet in half.
6. Serve hot.

Lunch Keto Meal Plan

In case you are confused about which recipes to include in your twenty-one days keto meal plan, this section has got all you need.

Asian Inspired Beef Salad

Total Prep & Cooking Time: Twenty-five minutes
Yields: Two servings
Nutrition Facts: Calories: 980.3 | Protein: 33.6g | Carbs: 5.7g| Fat: 98.6g | Fiber: 3.1g

Ingredients

For the sesame mayonnaise:

- Three-fourth cup of mayonnaise
- One tsp. of sesame oil
- Half tbsp. of lime juice
- Pepper and salt

For the beef:

- One tbsp. of each
  - Fish sauce
  - Olive oil
  - Ginger (grated)
- One tsp. of chili flakes
- Two-third pound of rib-eye steaks

For the salad:

- Three ounces of each
  - Lettuce
  - Cucumber
  - Cherry tomatoes
- Half red onion (sliced)
- Cilantro (chopped)
- One tsp. of sesame seeds
- Two scallions

Method:

1. Mix all the listed ingredients for the mayonnaise. Mix well. Keep aside.
2. Combine all the listed ingredients for the beef marinade in a large-sized bowl. Marinate the beef steaks for fifteen minutes.
3. Chop the veggies for the salad. Divide the salad among two plates.
4. Sear the steaks for five minutes on each side. Place the meat on a cutting board. Cut in thin slices.
5. Arrange the beef over the salad.
6. Serve immediately with a dollop of mayo mixture by the side.

Chicken Soup

Total Prep & Cooking Time: Thirty minutes
Yields: Eight servings
Nutrition Facts: Calories: 502.1 | Protein: 34.1g | Carbs: 3.8g| Fat: 42.4g | Fiber: 1.2g

Ingredients

Four ounces of butter
Two tbsps. of dried onion (minced)
Two stalks of celery (chopped)
Six ounces of mushrooms (sliced)
Two cloves of garlic (minced)
Eight cups of chicken stock
One carrot (sliced)
Two tsps. of parsley (dried)
One tsp. of salt
One-fourth of black pepper (ground)
One and a half rotisserie chicken (shredded)
Five ounces of green cabbage (sliced)

Method:

1. Melt the butter in a deep pot.
2. Add celery, dried onion, garlic, and mushrooms. SauteL for four minutes.
3. Add carrot, chicken stock, parsley, pepper, and salt. Simmer for two minutes.
4. Add the chicken along with cabbage. Simmer for twelve minutes.
5. Serve hot.

Smoked Salmon Plate

Total Prep & Cooking Time: Five minutes
Yields: Two servings
Nutrition Facts: Calories: 963.2 | Protein: 36.3g | Carbs: 1.1g| Fat: 98.7g | Fiber: 1.4g

Ingredients

Three-fourth pound of smoked salmon
One cup of mayonnaise
Two ounces of baby spinach
One tbsp. of olive oil
Half lime
Pepper and salt

Method:

1. Arrange spinach, salmon, lime wedge, and a dollop of mayo on serving plates.
2. Drizzle some olive oil from the top. Season with pepper and salt.
3. Serve immediately.

Keto Quesadillas

Total Prep & Cooking Time: Thirty minutes
Yields: Three servings
Nutrition Facts: Calories: 472.3 | Protein: 22.6g | Carbs: 4.9g| Fat: 42.3g | Fiber: 3.2g

Ingredients

For the tortillas:

- Two large eggs
- Two eggs whites
- Six ounces of cream cheese
- Half tsp. of salt
- Two tsps. of ground psyllium husk powder
- One tbsp. of coconut flour

For the filling:

- One tbsp. of butter
- Five ounces of Mexican cheese blend
- One ounce of baby spinach

Method:

1. Preheat your oven at two hundred degrees Celsius.
2. Beat the egg whites and eggs in a bowl. Add the cream cheese. Blend using an electric mixer.
3. Mix salt, coconut flour, and husk powder in a bowl.
4. Add the mixture of flour in the egg mixture. Mix well.
5. Spread the batter on a greased baking sheet. Bake for ten minutes.
6. Cut the tortilla rectangle into six small pieces.
7. Heat the butter in a pan.
8. Add one tortilla. Sprinkle with spinach and cheese. Top with another tortilla.
9. Fry for one minute on each side.

Cauliflower Soup and Crispy Pancetta Total Prep & Cooking Time: Twenty minutes Yields: Six servings

Nutrition Facts: Calories: 536.4 | Protein: 11.3g | Carbs: 5.6g| Fat: 54.6g | Fiber: 3.2g

Ingredients

Four cups of chicken stock
One pound of cauliflower
One tbsp. of butter
Seven ounces of cream cheese
One and a half tbsp. of Dijon mustard
Four ounces of butter
Pepper and salt
Seven ounces of pancetta (diced)
One tsp. of paprika powder
Three ounces of pecans

Method:

1. Cut the cauliflower into small florets.
2. Take a handful of the florets. Chop them into bite-size pieces.
3. SauteL pancetta and chopped florets in the butter for four minutes. Add paprika powder and nuts. Mix well.
4. Boil the florets of cauliflower in the stock. Add butter, mustard, and cream cheese.
5. Use an immersion blender for blending the soup. Blend until smooth. Add pepper and salt.
6. Divide the soup among serving bowls. Top with the fried mixture of pancetta.
7. Serve hot.

Dinner Keto Meal Plan

All the recipes that you will find in this section can help you bring about some serious changes in your health condition. Let's have a look at them.

Pesto Chicken Casserole With Cheese and Olives

Total Prep & Cooking Time: Forty-five minutes
Yields: Four servings
Nutrition Facts: Calories: 918.3 | Protein: 36.6g | Carbs: 5.7g| Fat: 94.3g | Fiber: 2.2g

Ingredients

- Two pounds of chicken breast
- Pepper and salt
- Two tbsps. of butter
- Five tbsps. of red pesto
- One and a half cup of whipping cream
- Three ounces of olives (pitted)
- Five ounces of feta cheese
- One clove of garlic (chopped)

Method:

1. Preheat your oven at two-hundred degrees Celsius.
2. Chop the chicken breast into bite-size cubes. Add pepper and salt.
3. Fry the chicken pieces in the butter.
4. Combine cream and red pesto in a bowl.
5. Arrange the cooked chicken pieces along with olives in a baking dish. Top with garlic and feta cheese. Add the mixture of pesto.
6. Bake for thirty minutes.
7. Serve hot.

Tortilla With Salsa and Ground Beef

Total Prep & Cooking Time: One hour and ten minutes
Yields: Four servings
Nutrition Facts: Calories: 820 | Protein: 41.3g | Carbs: 7.2g| Fat: 69.6g | Fiber: 12.3g

Ingredients

For the filling:

- Two tbsps. of olive oil
- One pound of beef (ground)
- Two tbsps. of tex-mex seasoning
- Half cup of water
- Pepper and salt

For the salsa:

- Two avocados (diced)
- One tomato (diced)
- Two tbsps. of lime juice
- One tbsp. of olive oil
- Half cup of cilantro (chopped)
- Pepper and salt

For serving:

- Six ounces of Mexican cheese (shredded)
- Three ounces of lettuce (shredded)
- Four low-carb tortillas

Method:

1. Take a large-sized non-stick pan and heat oil in it. Cook the beef for five minutes. Add water and seasoning. Simmer for five minutes. Add pepper and salt.
2. Combine the salsa ingredients in a bowl.
3. Arrange beef and salsa on the tortillas. Top with cheese.
4. Serve with lettuce by the side.

Keto Pork Chops With Garlic Butter and Green Beans

Total Prep & Cooking Time: Thirty minutes

Yields: Four servings

Nutrition Facts: Calories: 730.3 | Protein: 37.6g | Carbs: 5.8g| Fat: 63.6g | Fiber: 3.1g

Ingredients

For the garlic butter:

- Five ounces of butter
- Half tbsp. of garlic powder
- One tbsp. of each
  - Lemon juice
  - Parsley (dried)
- Pepper and salt

For the pork chops:

- Four pork chops
- Two ounces of butter
- One pound of green beans
- Pepper and salt

Method:

1. Combine the garlic butter ingredients in a bowl.
2. Use a sharp knife for making few cuts on the pork chops. Season with pepper and salt.
3. Melt the butter in an iron skillet. Add the chops. Fry for five minutes on each side. Remove the chops from the skillet.
4. Add the beans in the same skillet. Fry for two minutes. Season with pepper and salt.
5. Serve the chops with green beans and a spoonful of garlic butter on the top.

Fried Salmon With Cheese and Broccoli

Total Prep & Cooking Time: Thirty-five minutes
Yields: Four servings
Nutrition Facts: Calories: 682.6 | Protein: 45.9g | Carbs: 5.9g| Fat: 51.6g | Fiber: 3.3g

Ingredients

One pound of broccoli
Three ounces of butter
Pepper and salt
Five ounces of cheddar cheese (grated)
Two pounds of salmon
One lime

Method:

1. Preheat your oven at two hundred degrees Celsius.
2. Chop the broccoli into small florets. Simmer the florets in salted water for five minutes. Drain the florets and keep aside.
3. Arrange the florets in a baking dish. Add pepper and butter.
4. Sprinkle grated cheese from the top. Bake for twenty minutes.
5. Season the fish with pepper and salt.
6. Heat butter in an iron skillet. Fry the fish on each side for four minutes.
7. Serve the fish with broccoli by the side. Garnish with lime wedges.

Rib-Eye Steak With Roasted Veggies

Total Prep & Cooking Time: Forty minutes Yields: Four servings

Nutrition Facts: Calories: 797.6 | Protein: 42.1g | Carbs: 9.8g| Fat: 66.3g | Fiber: 4.1g

Ingredients

- One pound of broccoli
- One whole garlic
- Ten ounces of cherry tomatoes
- Three tbsps. of olive oil
- One tbsp. of thyme (dried)
- Two pounds of rib-eye steaks
- Pepper and salt

For the anchovy butter:

- One ounce of anchovies
- Five ounces of butter
- One tbsp. of lemon juice
- Pepper and salt

Method:

1. Start with the anchovy butter by chopping the anchovy fillets. Combine with butter, pepper, lemon juice, and salt.
2. Preheat your oven at two hundred degrees Celsius.
3. Slice the broccoli into florets. Separate the cloves of garlic.
4. Grease a baking pan with butter. Add the veggies. Drizzle some olive oil from the top. Roast in the oven for fifteen minutes.
5. Season the steaks with pepper, salt, and add some olive oil.
6. Fry the steaks in an iron skillet for five minutes on each side.
7. Take out the veggie pan and make some room for the steaks.
8. Add the steaks in the pan along with the veggies.
9. Roast for fifteen minutes.
10. Serve with a spoonful of anchovy butter on the top.

Snacks Keto Meal Plan

Snacks form an important part of everyday meals. The aim is to satisfy your cravings without opting for something unhealthy. Here are some tasty keto snack recipes for you that you can make in no time.

Keto Bread Twists

Total Prep & Cooking Time: Forty minutes
Yields: Ten servings
Nutrition Facts: Calories: 210.3 | Protein: 8.6g | Carbs: 1.1g| Fat: 18.3g | Fiber: 2.3g

Ingredients

- Half cup of almond flour
- One-fourth cup of coconut flour
- Half tsp. of salt
- One tsp. of baking powder
- One large egg (beaten)
- Two ounces of butter
- Seven ounces of cheese (shredded)
- One cup of green pesto
- One egg (for brushing)

Method:

1. Preheat your oven at one hundred and fifty degrees Celsius.
2. Mix all the dry listed ingredients along with the beaten egg.
3. Melt cheese and butter in a medium pot. Keep stirring until the batter becomes smooth.
4. Add the butter and cheese mixture to the dry ingredient mix. Mix well for making a firm dough.
5. Flatten the dough into a rectangle. Add green pesto on the top.
6. Cut the dough into strips of one-inch. Twist the strips. Arrange them on a baking pan. Brush the twisted strips with egg.
7. Bake for twenty minutes.

Burger Fat Bombs

Total Prep & Cooking Time: Thirty minutes
Yields: Ten servings
Nutrition Facts: Calories: 82.1 | Protein: 5g | Carbs: 0.2g| Fat: 7.2g | Fiber: 0.6g

Ingredients

- One pound of beef (ground)
- Cooking spray
- Half tsp. of garlic powder
- Kosher salt
- Black pepper (ground)
- Two tbsps. of butter (cut into twenty cubes)
- Two ounces of cheddar cheese (cut into twenty pieces)

Method:

1. Preheat your oven at one hundred and seventy degrees Celsius.
2. Use cooking spray for greasing a muffin tin.
3. Combine garlic powder, beef, pepper, and salt in a bowl.
4. Press one tsp. of the meat mixture into the base of each muffin cup. Add one cube of butter and top with one tsp. of meat. Add a piece of cheese on the top.
5. Bake for fifteen minutes.
6. Use a small knife for removing bombs.
7. Serve hot.

Crab Avocado Boats

Total Prep & Cooking Time: Twenty minutes
Yields: Four servings
Nutrition Facts: Calories: 330.6 | Protein: 31.1g | Carbs: 8.8g| Fat: 20.1g | Fiber: 5.3g

Ingredients

- Twelve ounces of crab meat
- One-third cup of Greek yogurt
- Half red onion (minced)
- Two tbsps. of chives (chopped)
- Three tbsps. of lemon juice
- Half tsp. of cayenne pepper
- Kosher salt
- One cup of cheddar cheese (shredded)
- Two avocados (halved, pitted)

Method:

1. Combine crab meat, yogurt, chives, red onion, cayenne, and lemon juice in a bowl. Add salt for seasoning.
2. Scoop out avocado pulp for making bowls. Add the scooped-out pulp in the mixture of crab.
3. Fill the avocado bowl with the mixture of crab. Add cheese from the top.
4. Broil for one minute.

Keto Taquitos

Total Prep & Cooking Time: Forty-five minutes
Yields: Six servings
Nutrition Facts: Calories: 229.6 | Protein: 18.2g | Carbs: 2.1g| Fat: 19.8g | Fiber: 0.3g

Ingredients

- Two tbsps. of olive oil
- Half onion (chopped)
- Four garlic cloves (minced)
- One tsp. of each
  - Chili powder
  - Cumin (ground)
- Two cups of each
  - Chicken shredded
  - Monterey jack cheese (shredded)
  - Cheddar cheese (shredded)
- Two-third cup of red enchilada sauce
- Four tbsps. of cilantro (chopped)
- Kosher salt

Method:

1. Preheat your oven at one hundred and seventy degrees Celsius.
2. Use parchment paper for lining two baking sheets.
3. Heat oil in an iron skillet. Add chopped onion and garlic. SauteL for three minutes. Sprinkle the spices over the garlic-onion mixture. Keep stirring for two minutes. Now it is time to add the chicken along with the enchilada sauce. Simmer the mixture for three minutes. Add cilantro. Keep aside.
4. Combine the cheeses in a bowl. Divide the cheese mixture into twelve equal three-inch piles on the baking sheets. Bake for ten minutes.
5. Let the taquito shells cool down for four minutes.
6. Add the chicken mixture in the shells and roll.
7. Serve immediately.

Cheese, Ham, and Egg Roll-Ups

Total Prep & Cooking Time: Thirty-five minutes
Yields: Ten servings
Nutrition Facts: Calories: 415.3 | Protein: 37.6g | Carbs: 5.6g| Fat: 27.2g | Fiber: 1.2g

Ingredients

- Ten large eggs
- Two tsps. of garlic powder
- Kosher salt
- Black pepper (ground)
- Two tbsps. of butter
- Two cups of cheddar cheese (shredded)
- One cup of baby spinach
- Half cup of tomatoes (chopped)
- Two slices of ham

Method:

1. Beat the eggs with pepper, garlic powder, and salt in a mixing bowl.
2. Melt the butter in a skillet. Add the eggs. Scramble and cook for four minutes. Add the cheese, tomatoes, and spinach.
3. Place two ham slices on a cutting board. Add one tbsp. of the egg mixture. Roll the ham slices.
4. Arrange the rolled ham slices in a baking tray. Bake for five minutes.
5. Serve hot.

Chapter 5: Easy Keto Breakfast Recipes

Here are some tasty breakfast recipes for you with which you can start your day with a kick.

French Omelet

Total Prep & Cooking Time: Twenty minutes
Yields: Two servings
Nutrition Facts: Calories: 189 | Protein: 22.3g | Carbs: 3.6g| Fat: 10.9g | Fiber: 0.1g

Ingredients

- Two large eggs
- Four egg whites
- One-fourth cup of milk
- One-eighth tsp. of each
  - Pepper
  - Salt
- One cup of ham (cooked)
- One tbsp. of each
  - Green pepper (chopped)
  - Onion (chopped)
- Half cup of cheddar cheese (shredded)

Method:

1. Whisk the first five listed ingredients.
2. Use cooking spray for greasing a skillet. Place the skillet over medium flame. Add the mixture of eggs.
3. Cook for two minutes.
4. Top with the remaining ingredients. Fold the egg in half.
5. Cut the omelet in half. Serve immediately.

Sage Sausage Patty

Total Prep & Cooking Time: One hour and fifteen minutes
Yields: Eight servings
Nutrition Facts: Calories: 160.3 | Protein: 14.6g | Carbs: 1.2g| Fat: 12.3g | Fiber: 0.3g

Ingredients

One pound of pork (ground)
Three-fourth cup of cheddar cheese (ground)
One-fourth cup of buttermilk
One tbsp. of onion (chopped)
Two tsps. of sage
Three-fourth tsp. of each

- Pepper
- Salt

Half tsp. of each

- Oregano (dried)
- Garlic powder

Method:

1. Combine the listed ingredients either in a bowl or in a food processor.
2. Shape the mixture into eight equal patties of half-inch. Refrigerate the patties for one hour.
3. Heat oil in an iron skillet. Cook the patties on each side for six minutes.
4. Serve hot.

Feta Frittata

Total Prep & Cooking Time: Thirty minutes
Yields: Two servings
Nutrition Facts: Calories: 205.3 | Protein: 19.3g | Carbs: 6.7g| Fat: 12.5g | Fiber: 3.6g

Ingredients

- One green onion (sliced)
- One clove of garlic (minced)
- Two large eggs
- Half cup of egg substitute
- Four tbsps. of feta cheese (crumbled)
- One-third cup of plum tomato (chopped)
- Four slices of avocado (peeled)
- Two tbsps. of sour cream

Method:

1. Heat oil in an iron skillet. Add garlic and onion. SauteL for three minutes.
2. Combine egg substitute, eggs, and three tbsps. of feta cheese in a bowl. Add the mixture of eggs to the skillet.
3. Cook for six minutes.
4. Sprinkle remaining feta and tomato from the top.
5. Cover and cook for two minutes.
6. Let the egg stand for five minutes.
7. Serve with sour cream and avocado.

Ham Steak With Bacon, Mushrooms, and Gruyere

Total Prep & Cooking Time: Thirty-five minutes
Yields: Four servings
Nutrition Facts: Calories: 356.3 | Protein: 35.4g | Carbs: 5.1g| Fat: 23.2g | Fiber: 1.1g

Ingredients

- Two tbsps. of butter
- Half pound of mushrooms (sliced)
- One shallot (chopped)
- Two cloves of garlic (minced)
- One-eighth tsp. of black pepper (ground)
- One boneless ham steak (cooked, cut in four equal pieces)
- One cup of gruyere cheese (shredded)
- Four strips of bacon (cooked, crumbled)
- One tbsp. of parsley (minced)

Method:

1. Heat butter in a large iron skillet. Add shallot and mushrooms. Cook the mixture for six minutes. Mix garlic and pepper. SauteL for two minutes. Keep aside.
2. Cook the ham in the same skillet. Add bacon and cheese. Cook for two minutes.
3. Serve the ham with the mushroom mixture from the top.

Mushroom-Mascarpone Frittata

Total Prep & Cooking Time: Forty-five minutes
Yields: Six servings
Nutrition Facts: Calories: 469.3 | Protein: 18.7g | Carbs: 5.7g| Fat: 45.4g | Fiber: 1.6g

Ingredients

- Eight large eggs
- One-third cup of whipping cream
- Half cup of Romano cheese (grated)
- Two tsps. of salt
- Five tbsps. of olive oil
- Three-fourth pound of fresh mushrooms (sliced)
- One onion (sliced)
- Two tbsps. of basil (minced)
- Two cloves of garlic (minced)
- One-eighth tsp. of pepper
- Eight ounces of mascarpone cheese

Method:

1. Whisk together cream, eggs, one-fourth cup of Romano cheese, and salt in a bowl.
2. Heat two tbsps. of oil in a pan. Add mushrooms and onion. SauteL for two minutes. Add garlic, basil, along with pepper. Stir for one minute. Remove from heat. Add Romano cheese and mascarpone cheese.
3. Heat one tbsp. of oil in the same pan. Add half mixture of eggs in the pan. Keep cooking for seven minutes. Repeat with the remaining egg mixture.
4. Place one egg frittata on a plate. Add the mixture of mushrooms. Spread properly.
5. Add the other layer of frittata.
6. Cut in wedges.
7. Serve immediately.

Broccoli Quiche Cups

Total Prep & Cooking Time: Twenty-five minutes
Yields: Six servings
Nutrition Facts: Calories: 292.3 | Protein: 17.6g | Carbs: 3.6g| Fat: 25.4g | Fiber: 0.7g

Ingredients

- One cup of broccoli (chopped)
- One and a half cup of pepper jack cheese (shredded)
- Six large eggs
- Three-fourth cup of whipping cream
- Half cup of bacon bits
- One shallot (minced)
- One-fourth tsp. of each
  - Pepper
  - Salt

Method:

1. Preheat your oven at one-hundred and seventy degrees Celsius.
2. Divide the cheese and chopped broccoli among twelve greased muffin cups.
3. Combine the remaining ingredients in a bowl. Divide the prepared mixture among the cups.
4. Bake the quiche cups for twenty minutes.
5. Serve immediately.

Savory Chicken Sausage-Apple

Total Prep & Cooking Time: Twenty-five minutes
Yields: Four servings
Nutrition Facts: Calories: 93.6 | Protein: 9.9g | Carbs: 3.2g| Fat: 6.5g | Fiber: 1.2g

Ingredients

One tart apple (peeled, diced)
Two tsps. of poultry seasoning
One tsp. of salt
One-fourth tsp. of pepper
One pound of chicken (ground)

Method:

1. Take a large bowl. Mix the first four ingredients. Crumble the chicken over the apple mixture. Combine well. Shape the mixture into eight equal patties of three-inch.
2. Heat oil in an iron skillet.
3. Cook the apple-chicken patties for six minutes on each side.
4. Serve hot.

Manchego and Shiitake Scramble

Total Prep & Cooking Time: Twenty-five minutes
Yields: Eight servings
Nutrition Facts: Calories: 270.6 | Protein: 12.1g | Carbs: 3.4g| Fat: 23.6g | Fiber: 1.1g

Ingredients

- Two tbsps. of olive oil
- Half cup of each
  - Sweet red pepper (diced)
  - Onion (diced)
- Two cups of shiitake mushrooms (sliced)
- One tsp. of prepared horseradish
- Eight large eggs (beaten)
- One cup of each
  - Whipping cream
  - Manchego cheese (shredded)
- Half tsp. of each
  - Pepper (ground)
  - Kosher salt

Method:

1. Heat one tbsp. of oil in an iron skillet. Add red pepper and onion. Cook for three minutes. Cook the mixture for four minutes after adding the mushrooms along with horseradish. Stir for two minutes.
2. Whisk the remaining ingredients in a bowl with some olive oil. Pour the mixture into the skillet.
3. Cook and scramble the eggs for four minutes.
4. Serve hot.

Three-Cheese Quiche

Total Prep & Cooking Time: One hour and ten minutes
Yields: Six servings
Nutrition Facts: Calories: 448.3 | Protein: 21.2g | Carbs: 5.2g| Fat: 38.6g | Fiber: 0.2g

Ingredients

- Seven large eggs
- Five egg yolks
- One cup of each
  - Whipping cream
  - Half and half cream
  - Mozzarella cheese (shredded)
- Three-fourth cup of cheddar cheese (shredded)
- Half cup of Swiss cheese (shredded)
- Two tbsps. of sun-dried tomatoes
- One and half tsp. of seasoning blend
- One-fourth tsp. of basil (dried)

Method:

1. Preheat your oven at one hundred and fifty degrees Celsius.
2. Combine egg yolks, eggs, whipping cream, mozzarella cheese, half and half cream, half cup of cheddar cheese, tomatoes, Swiss cheese, basil, and seasoning blend in a greased pie dish. Sprinkle the remaining cheddar cheese from the top.
3. Bake for fifty minutes.
4. Let the quiche sit for ten minutes.
5. Cut in triangles and serve.

Breakfast Turkey Sausage

Total Prep & Cooking Time: Twenty minutes

Yields: Eight servings

Nutrition Facts: Calories: 87.6 | Protein: 11.3g | Carbs: 0.2g| Fat: 7.5g | Fiber: 0.1g

Ingredients

One pound of lean turkey (ground)

Three-fourth tsp. of salt

Half tsp. of rubbed sage

One-fourth tsp. of ginger (ground)

One-third tsp. of pepper (ground)

Method:

1. Crumble the turkey meat in a large bowl. Add sage, salt, ginger, and pepper. Shape the mixture into eight equal patties of two-inch.
2. Grease an iron skillet with oil.
3. Add the patties. Cook for six minutes on each side.

No-Bread Breakfast Sandwich

Total Prep & Cooking Time: Fifteen minutes
Yields: Two servings
Nutrition Facts: Calories: 356.3 | Protein: 20.3g | Carbs: 2.1g| Fat: 31.1g | Fiber: 0.2g

Ingredients

- Two tbsps. of butter
- Four large eggs
- Pepper and salt
- One ounce of deli ham (smoked)
- Two ounces of cheddar cheese (cut in slices)
- Few drops of Tabasco

Method:

1. Heat the butter in an iron skillet. Add the eggs. Fry each side for two minutes. Add pepper and salt.
2. Take a fried egg. Add ham and cheese. Top with another fried egg.
3. Repeat for the other fried eggs.
4. Place the sandwich in the pan for one minute.
5. Sprinkle some Tabasco from the top.
6. Serve hot.

Baked Eggs

Total Prep & Cooking Time: Twenty minutes
Yields: One serving
Nutrition Facts: Calories: 497.6 | Protein: 42.1g | Carbs: 2.1g| Fat: 34.5g | Fiber: 0.3g

Ingredients

- Three ounces of beef (ground)
- Two large eggs
- Two ounces of cheese (shredded)

Method:

1. Preheat your oven at two hundred degrees Celsius.
2. Arrange the ground beef as the base in a baking dish.
3. Make two holes in the beef base. Crack the eggs in the holes.
4. Sprinkle cheese from the top.
5. Bake for fifteen minutes.
6. Let the baked eggs sit for five minutes.

Cured Salmon With Chives and Scrambled Eggs

Total Prep & Cooking Time: Fifteen minutes
Yields: Two servings
Nutrition Facts: Calories: 730.2 | Protein: 49.6g | Carbs: 2.1g| Fat: 61.3g | Fiber: 0.1g

Ingredients

Two large eggs
Two tbsps. of butter
One-fourth cup of whipping cream
One tbsp. of chives (chopped)
Two ounces of cured salmon
Pepper and salt

Method:

1. Begin with whisking the eggs in a bowl.
2. Heat the butter in a pan. Add the eggs. Add the cream. Stir for three minutes.
3. Simmer for five minutes. Keep stirring for making the eggs creamy.
4. Add salt, chopped chives, and pepper.
5. Serve the eggs with cured salmon.

Eggs Benedict on Avocados

Total Prep & Cooking Time: Twenty minutes
Yields: Four servings
Nutrition Facts: Calories: 523.6 | Protein: 17.6g | Carbs: 3.1g| Fat: 49.3g | Fiber: 7.1g

Ingredients

For the hollandaise:

- Three egg yolks
- One tbsp. of lemon juice
- Pepper and salt
- Eight tbsps. of butter (unsalted)

For the eggs:

- Two avocados (pitted, skinned)
- Four large eggs
- Five ounces of salmon (smoked)

Method:

1. Add the butter in a bowl. Microwave for twenty seconds.
2. Add lemon juice and egg yolks. Use a hand blender for properly blending the mixture. Keep blending until a white layer forms. Add pepper and salt. Blend for two minutes.
3. Boil water in a saucepan. Crack the eggs in a small cup. Crack one egg at a time. Slide the eggs gently into the water. Cook for four minutes.
4. Cut the avocados in half. Add an egg on top of each avocado slice. Add hollandaise sauce from the top.
5. Add smoked salmon by the side.
6. Serve immediately.

Keto Chaffles

Total Prep & Cooking Time: Ten minutes

Yields: Four servings

Nutrition Facts: Calories: 332.3 | Protein: 23.2g | Carbs: 1.9g| Fat: 28.6g | Fiber: 0.2g

Ingredients

- One ounce of butter (melted)
- Four large eggs
- Eight ounces of mozzarella cheese (shredded)
- Four tbsps. of almond flour
- One pinch of salt

Method:

1. Preheat a waffle maker.
2. Mix all the ingredients that has been listed in a mixing bowl. Combine well.
3. Use butter for greasing the waffle maker.
4. Add one spoonful of the batter in the waffle maker. Close the waffle maker. Cook for six minutes.
5. Serve immediately with toppings of your choice.

Asparagus and Smoked Salmon Frittata

Total Prep & Cooking Time: Forty minutes
Yields: Four servings
Nutrition Facts: Calories: 511.3 | Protein: 28.9g | Carbs: 3.4g| Fat: 44.3g | Fiber: 1.2g

Ingredients

- Eight large eggs
- One cup of whipping cream
- One tsp. of salt
- Half tsp. of pepper
- One and a half tsp. of dill (dried)
- Four ounces of mozzarella cheese (shredded)
- Two ounces of parmesan cheese (shredded)
- Half ounce of butter
- Three and a half ounces of smoked salmon
- Two and a half ounces of green asparagus

Method:

1. Preheat your oven at one hundred and fifty degrees Celsius.
2. Combine eggs, seasonings, cream, half of the mozzarella cheese, and parmesan cheese in a large bowl.
3. Use butter for greasing a baking dish.
4. Add chunks of smoked salmon all over the base of the baking dish.
5. Arrange the spears of asparagus over the base of salmon.
6. Pour the mixture of eggs over the asparagus. Sprinkle mozzarella from the top.
7. Bake the frittata for thirty minutes.

Vegetable Keto Scramble

Total Prep & Cooking Time: Twenty minutes

Yields: One serving

Nutrition Facts: Calories: 410.3 | Protein: 28.2g | Carbs: 3.6g| Fat: 32.3g | Fiber: 1.1g

Ingredients

One tbsp. of butter
One ounce of mushrooms (sliced)
Three large eggs
One and a half ounces of red bell pepper (diced)
Pepper and salt
Half ounce of parmesan cheese (shredded)
Half a scallion (chopped)

Method:

1. Melt the butter in an iron skillet. Add red peppers and mushrooms. Season with pepper and salt. Cook for four minutes.
2. Break the eggs into the skillet directly. Stir all the ingredients for combining.
3. Cook for four minutes. Keep stirring for keeping the eggs soft.
4. Serve with scallions and parmesan cheese from the top.

French Pancakes

Total Prep & Cooking Time: Fifteen minutes
Yields: Four servings
Nutrition Facts: Calories: 695 | Protein: 14.6g | Carbs: 3.3g| Fat: 67.8g | Fiber: 4.2g

Ingredients

- Eight large eggs
- Two cups of whipping cream
- Half cup of water
- One-fourth tsp. of salt
- Two tbsps. of psyllium husk powder
- Three ounces of butter

Method:

1. Combine cream, eggs, salt, and water in a bowl. Use a hand blender for proper mixing.
2. Add psyllium husk powder. Keep mixing. Let the batter rest for ten minutes.
3. Add butter in a pan. Fry the pancakes for four minutes on each side.
4. Serve hot.

Lettuce Wraps

Total Prep & Cooking Time: Twenty minutes
Yields: Two servings
Nutrition Facts: Calories: 580.6 | Protein: 12.3g | Carbs: 3.9g| Fat: 57.6g | Fiber: 4.3g

Ingredients

- Six ounces of bacon slices
- Three tbsps. of mayonnaise
- Two ounces of lettuce
- Half an avocado
- One tomato (sliced)
- Pepper and salt

Method:

1. Fry the slices of bacon in an iron skillet. Fry for five minutes. Let the bacon slices sit for five minutes. Cut the strips in half.
2. Arrange the lettuce leaves on a cutting board. Squeeze lemon juice on the leaves. Add half slice of tomato, one slice of avocado, and three halves of bacon slices. Add pepper and salt.
3. Wrap the lettuce leaves.
4. Serve immediately.

Deviled Eggs

Total Prep & Cooking Time: Fifteen minutes
Yields: Four servings
Nutrition Facts: Calories: 167.3 | Protein: 7.6g | Carbs: 0.4g| Fat: 14.6g | Fiber: 0.2g

Ingredients

Four large eggs
One tsp. of Tabasco
One-fourth cup of mayonnaise
One pinch of herbal salt
Eight shrimps (peeled, cooked)
Dried dill

Method:

1. Boil the eggs in salted water. Boil for ten minutes.
2. Transfer the eggs to an ice bath. Let the eggs sit for two minutes. Peel the eggs.
3. Cut the eggs in half. Remove the yolks.
4. Arrange the eggs whites on a large plate.
5. Combine the yolks, mayonnaise, herbal salt, and Tabasco in one bowl. Use fork for mashing the ingredients.
6. Scoop two tsps. of the mixture of egg yolks into the egg whites. Top with the cooked shrimps.
7. Garnish with dill.
8. Serve immediately.

Keto Breakfast Cereal

Total Prep & Cooking Time: Forty minutes
Yields: Four servings
Nutrition Facts: Calories: 357.6 | Protein: 10.3g | Carbs: 9.3g| Fat: 29.6g | Fiber: 5.6g

Ingredients

- One cup of each
  - Walnuts (chopped)
  - Almonds (chopped)
  - Coconut flakes
- One-fourth cup of sesame seeds
- Two tbsps. of each
  - Chia seeds
  - Flax seeds
- Half tsp. of clove (ground)
- Two tsps. of ground cinnamon
- One tsp. of vanilla extract
- One-third tsp. of kosher salt
- One large egg white
- One-fourth cup of coconut oil (melted)

Method:

1. Preheat your oven at one hundred and fifty degrees Celsius.
2. Use cooking spray for greasing a medium baking tray.
3. Combine walnuts, almonds, flax seeds, coconut flakes, sesame seeds, and chia seeds in a bowl. Add cinnamon, cloves, salt, and vanilla extract. Mix well.
4. Beat the egg white in a small-sized bowl until foamy. Add it to the cereal mix.
5. Add the oil and mix.
6. Pour the cereal mix on the baking tray. Evenly spread out the cereal mix.
7. Bake for twenty minutes.
8. Let the cereal mix cool down completely and serve.

Breakfast Cups

Total Prep & Cooking Time: Forty minutes
Yields: Six servings
Nutrition Facts: Calories: 210.1 | Protein: 7.6g | Carbs: 1.2g| Fat: 53.4g | Fiber: 1.1g

Ingredients

- Two pounds of pork (ground)
- One tbsp. of thyme (chopped)
- Two cloves of garlic (minced)
- Half tsp. of each
  - Cumin (ground)
  - Paprika
- One tsp. of kosher salt
- Black pepper (ground)
- Three cups of spinach (chopped)
- One cup of white cheddar cheese (shredded)
- Twelve large eggs
- One tbsp. of chives (chopped)

Method:

1. Preheat your oven at two hundred degrees Celsius.
2. Combine thyme, pork, paprika, garlic, salt, and cumin in a bowl. Add pepper for seasoning.
3. Grease a muffin tin with cooking spray.
4. Add one handful of the pork mixture into each cup of the muffin tray. Press the mixture for forming a cup. Arrange spinach and cheese among the meat cups.
5. Crack one egg over each cup. Season with pepper and salt.
6. Bake for twenty-five minutes.
7. Garnish with chopped chives.
8. Serve hot.

Omelet Stuffed Pepper

Total Prep & Cooking Time: One hour
Yields: Four servings
Nutrition Facts: Calories: 150.3 | Protein: 10.2g | Carbs: 6.8g| Fat: 9.7g | Fiber: 1.9g

Ingredients

Two bell peppers (halved, remove the seeds)
Eight large eggs (beaten)
One-fourth cup of milk
Four bacon slices (cooked, crumbled)
One cup of cheddar cheese (shredded)
Two tbsps. of chives (chopped)
Black pepper (ground)
Kosher salt

Method:

1. Heat your oven at two hundred degrees Celsius.
2. Arrange the peppers in a baking dish with the cut side up.
3. Add some water in the dish. Bake for five minutes.
4. Combine milk and eggs in a bowl. Add cheese, bacon, and chives. Add pepper and salt for seasoning.
5. Divide the egg mixture among the peppers. Bake for forty minutes.
6. Garnish with chives.
7. Serve hot.

Brussels Sprouts Hash

Total Prep & Cooking Time: Forty minutes
Yields: Four servings
Nutrition Facts: Calories: 402.1 | Protein: 22.1g | Carbs: 5.6g| Fat: 31.2g | Fiber: 4.6g

Ingredients

Six bacon slices (cut in one-inch piece)
Half onion (chopped)
One pound of Brussels sprouts (trimmed, quartered)
Kosher salt
Black pepper (ground)
One-fourth tsp. of red pepper flakes
Two cloves of garlic (minced)
Four large eggs

Method:

1. Cook the bacon pieces in an iron skillet until crispy. Keep aside.
2. Add Brussels sprouts and onion to the skillet. Add pepper, red pepper flakes, and salt. Cook for five minutes.
3. Add two tbsps. of water. Cover and cook for five minutes. Add the garlic. Cook for one minute.
4. Make four holes in the Brussels sprouts hash. Crack the eggs in the holes. Add pepper and salt.
5. Cover and cook for five minutes.
6. Garnish with cooked bits of bacon.
7. Serve hot.

Breakfast Stack

Total Prep & Cooking Time: Thirty minutes

Yields: Three servings

Nutrition Facts: Calories: 612.8 | Protein: 37.8g | Carbs: 9.3g| Fat: 53.4g | Fiber: 6.8g

Ingredients

- Three patties of breakfast sausage
- One avocado (mashed)
- Black pepper (ground)
- Kosher salt
- Three large eggs
- Chopped chives (to garnish)

Method:

1. Prepare the breakfast sausage patties following the instructions on the box.
2. Add the mashed avocado on the sausage patties. Add pepper and salt.
3. Heat oil in a skillet. Crack the eggs. Season with pepper and salt. Cook for three minutes.
4. Add the eggs over the sausage patties.
5. Garnish with chopped chives.
6. Serve hot.

Cauliflower Benedict

Total Prep & Cooking Time: Thirty minutes

Yields: Two servings

Nutrition Facts: Calories: 269.3 | Protein: 17.6g | Carbs: 6.3g| Fat: 17.3g | Fiber: 1.3g

Ingredients

For the patties:

- Half head of cauliflower
- One large egg
- Half tsp. of cornstarch
- One cup of cheddar cheese (shredded)
- Black pepper (ground)
- One tbsp. of olive oil

For the eggs:

- Two large eggs

For the sauce:

- Four large egg yolks
- Two tbsps. of lemon juice
- One tbsp. of butter (melted)
- Half tsp. of cayenne pepper
- Salt

For the assembly:

- Two slices of bacon (warmed)
- Paprika (to garnish)
- Chives (chopped, to garnish)

Method:

1. Grate the cauliflower. Combine eggs and grated cauliflower in a bowl. Add salt, cornstarch, and cheese. Mix well.
2. Make patties from the mixture.
3. Heat oil in an iron skillet. Add the patties. Cook for five minutes. Flip and cook for five minutes.
4. Start poaching the eggs in a large pot of hot water. Cook for three minutes.
5. Heat the egg yolks in a double boiler. Add the lemon juice and keep whisking. Add butter, salt, and cayenne. Mix well.
6. Serve the cauliflower patties and top with bacon, poached eggs, and sauce.
7. Garnish with chives and paprika.

Bacon Breakfast Tacos

Total Prep & Cooking Time: One hour
Yields: Four servings
Nutrition Facts: Calories: 395.6 | Protein: 24.2g | Carbs: 4.1g| Fat: 31.1g | Fiber: 2.6g

Ingredients

- Sixteen bacon slices (halved)
- Black pepper (ground)
- Six large eggs
- One tbsp. of each
  - Butter
  - Whole milk
- Kosher salt
- Two tbsps. of chives (chopped)
- One-fourth cup of Monterey jack cheese
- One avocado (sliced)

Method:

1. For the taco shells: preheat your oven at two hundred degrees Celsius.
2. Line a baking sheet with the help of aluminum foil.
3. Prepare bacon weaves with eight halves of bacon for each. Make four weaves. Add pepper and salt. Bake for thirty minutes.
4. Trim the sides of the taco shells for making rounds.
5. Whisk milk and eggs in a bowl.
6. Melt the butter in an iron skillet. Add the egg mixture. Scramble the eggs for three minutes. Add pepper and salt.
7. Add scrambled eggs in the taco shells. Add avocado slices and sprinkle cheese from the top.
8. Serve immediately.

Loaded Cauliflower Bake

Total Prep & Cooking Time: One hour and fifteen minutes
Yields: Six servings
Nutrition Facts: Calories: 393.6 | Protein: 27.2g | Carbs: 9.1g| Fat: 28.7g | Fiber: 3.2g

Ingredients

- One cauliflower
- Eight bacon slices (chopped)
- Ten large eggs
- Two cloves of garlic (minced)
- One cup of milk
- Two tsps. of paprika
- Kosher salt
- Two cups of cheddar cheese (shredded)
- Black pepper (ground)
- Two green onions (sliced)

Method:

1. Preheat your oven at one hundred and fifty degrees Celsius.
2. Grate the cauliflower.
3. Cook the bacon slices in an iron skillet for eight minutes.
4. Combine milk, eggs, paprika, and garlic in a bowl. Add pepper and salt.
5. Transfer grated cauliflower to a large baking dish. Top with cheddar cheese, green onions, and bacon. Pour over the mixture of eggs.
6. Bake for forty minutes.
7. Serve hot.

Chapter 6: Easy Keto Lunch Recipes

In this chapter, you will find some tasty keto lunch recipes that you can include in your diet plan without any worries. Let's have a look at them.

Turkey and Cream Cheese Sauce

Total Prep & Cooking Time: Twenty-five minutes
Yields: Five servings
Nutrition Facts: Calories: 810.3 | Protein: 47.6g | Carbs: 6.9g| Fat: 68.6g | Fiber: 0.6g

Ingredients

- Two tbsps. of butter
- Two pounds of turkey breast
- Two cups of whipping cream
- Seven ounces of cream cheese
- One tbsp. of tamari soy sauce
- Pepper and salt
- One and a half ounces of small capers

Method:

1. Preheat your oven at one hundred and seventy degrees Celsius.
2. Melt half butter in an iron skillet.
3. Season the breast of turkey with pepper and salt. Fry for five minutes.
4. Place the skillet in the oven. Bake for ten minutes.
5. Add the drippings of turkey in a pan. Add cream cheese and whipping cream. Simmer the mixture. Add pepper, soy sauce, and salt.
6. SauteL the small capers in remaining butter.
7. Slice the turkey.
8. Serve with fried capers and cream cheese sauce.

Baked Salmon and Pesto

Total Prep & Cooking Time: Twenty minutes
Yields: Four servings
Nutrition Facts: Calories: 1010.2 | Protein: 51.6g | Carbs: 3.1g| Fat: 87.6g | Fiber: 0.7g

Ingredients

For the green sauce:

- Four tbsps. of green pesto
- One cup of mayonnaise
- Half cup of Greek yogurt
- Pepper and salt

For the salmon:

- Two pounds of salmon
- Four tbsps. of green pesto
- Pepper and salt

Method:

1. Place the fillets of salmon on a greased baking dish with the skin side down. Add pesto on top. Add pepper and salt.
2. Bake at two hundred degrees Celsius for thirty minutes.
3. Combine all the listed ingredients for the green sauce in a bowl.
4. Serve the baked salmon with green sauce on top.

Keto Chicken With Butter and Lemon

Total Prep & Cooking Time: Two hours and ten minutes

Yields: Four servings

Nutrition Facts: Calories: 980.3 | Protein: 57.2g | Carbs: 0.4g| Fat: 81.3g | Fiber: 0.1g

Ingredients

- Three pounds of a whole chicken
- Pepper and salt
- Two tsps. of barbecue seasoning rub (dry)
- Five ounces of butter (sliced)
- One lemon (cut in wedges)
- Two onions (cut in wedges)
- One-fourth cup of water
- One tsp. of butter (to grease)

Method:

1. Preheat your oven at one hundred and seventy degrees Celsius.
2. Use butter for greasing a deep baking dish.
3. Season the chicken with pepper, salt, and barbecue rub. Place the chicken in the greased baking dish.
4. Arrange lemon wedges and onions surrounding the chicken. Add slices of butter on the chicken.
5. Bake for one hour and thirty minutes. Make sure you baste the whole chicken with the drippings occasionally.
6. Cut the chicken in pieces.
7. Serve hot.

Garlic Chicken

Total Prep & Cooking Time: One hour and ten minutes
Yields: Four servings
Nutrition Facts: Calories: 540.3 | Protein: 41.3g | Carbs: 3.1g| Fat: 38.6g | Fiber: 1.6g

Ingredients

Two ounces of butter
Two pounds of chicken drumsticks
Pepper and salt
One lemon (juiced)
Two tbsps. of olive oil
Seven cloves of garlic (sliced)
Half cup of parsley (chopped)

Method:

1. Preheat your oven at two hundred and fifty degrees Celsius.
2. Arrange the pieces of chicken in a greased baking dish. Add pepper and salt.
3. Add olive oil along with lemon juice over the chicken. Sprinkle parsley and garlic on top.
4. Bake for forty minutes.
5. Serve hot.

Salmon Skewers Wrapped With Prosciutto

Total Prep & Cooking Time: Thirty-five minutes
Yields: Four servings
Nutrition Facts: Calories: 670.5 | Protein: 27.2g | Carbs: 1.2g| Fat: 61.6g | Fiber: 0.3g

Ingredients

- One-fourth cup of basil (chopped)
- One pound of salmon
- One pinch of black pepper (ground)
- Four ounces of prosciutto (sliced)
- One tbsp. of olive oil
- Eight skewers (wooden)

Method:

1. Start by soaking the skewers in a bowl of water.
2. Cut the salmon fillets length-wise. Thread the salmon on the soaked skewers.
3. Coat the skewers in pepper and basil.
4. Wrap the slices of prosciutto all around the salmon.
5. Heat oil in a grill pan. Grill the skewers for four minutes.
6. Serve hot.

Buffalo Drumsticks and Chili Aioli

Total Prep & Cooking Time: Fifty minutes
Yields: Four servings
Nutrition Facts: Calories: 567.8 | Protein: 41.3g | Carbs: 2.2g| Fat: 43.2g | Fiber: 1.1g

Ingredients

For the chili aioli:

- Half cup of mayonnaise
- One tbsp. of smoked paprika powder
- One clove of garlic (minced)

For the chicken:

- Two pounds of chicken drumsticks
- Two tbsps. of each
  - White wine vinegar
  - Olive oil
- One tbsp. of tomato paste
- One tsp. of each
  - Salt
  - Paprika powder
  - Tabasco

Method:

1. Preheat your oven at two hundred degrees Celsius.
2. Combine the listed marinade ingredients. Marinate the chicken drumsticks for ten minutes.
3. Coat a baking tray with oil.
4. Arrange the chicken drumsticks in the tray. Bake for forty minutes.
5. Combine the listed ingredients for the chili aioli in a bowl.
6. Serve the drumsticks with chili aioli by the side.

Slow Cooked Roasted Pork and Creamy Gravy

Total Prep & Cooking Time: Eight hours and forty minutes
Yields: Six servings
Nutrition Facts: Calories: 586.9 | Protein: 27.9g | Carbs: 2.6g| Fat: 50.3g | Fiber: 1.5g

Ingredients

For the creamy gravy:

Two cups of whipping cream
Roast juice

For the pork:

Two pounds of pork roast
Half tbsp. of salt
One bay leaf
Five black peppercorns
Three cups of water
Two tsps. of thyme (dried)
Two cloves of garlic
Two ounces of ginger
One tbsp. of each
- Paprika powder
- Olive oil

One-third tsp. of black pepper (ground)

Method:

1. Preheat your oven at one hundred degrees Celsius.
2. Add the meat in a baking dish. Add salt. Add water for covering one-third of the meat. Add peppercorns, thyme, and bay leaf. Place the meat in the oven for eight hours. Cover the dish with aluminum foil.
3. Take out the meat from the oven. Reserve the juices from the dish.
4. Increase the temperature of the oven to two hundred degrees Celsius.
5. Grate ginger and garlic in a bowl. Add pepper, herbs, and oil. Rub the herb mixture on the meat.
6. Roast the meat for fifteen minutes.
7. Cut the roasted meat in slices.
8. Strain the meat juices in a bowl. Boil for reducing it by half.
9. Add the cream. Mix well. Simmer for twenty minutes.
10. Serve the roasted pork with creamy gravy from the top.

Bacon-Wrapped Meatloaf

Total Prep & Cooking Time: One hour twenty-five minutes
Yields: Four servings
Nutrition Facts: Calories: 1020.3 | Protein: 46.7g | Carbs: 5.6g| Fat: 88.9g | Fiber: 1.2g

Ingredients

For the meatloaf:

- Two tbsps. of butter
- One onion (chopped)
- Two pounds of beef (ground)
- Half cup of whipping cream
- Two ounces of cheese (shredded)
- One large egg (beaten)
- One tbsp. of oregano (dried)
- One tsp. of salt
- Half tsp. of black pepper (ground)
- Seven ounces of bacon (sliced)

For the gravy:

- One and a half cup of whipping cream
- Half tbsp. of tamari soy sauce

Method:

1. Preheat your oven at two hundred degrees Celsius.
2. Melt the butter in a pan. Add the onion. Cook for four minutes. Keep aside.
3. Combine onion, ground meat, and the remaining ingredients in a large bowl. Do not mix the bacon.
4. Make a firm loaf. Add the meatloaf in an oil-greased baking dish. Use bacon strips for wrapping the loaf.
5. Bake the meatloaf for forty-five minutes.
6. Add the juices from the baking dish in a pan. Add the cream and boil. Simmer for ten minutes. Add the soy sauce.
7. Slice the meatloaf. Serve with gravy from the top.

Lamb Chops and Herb Butter

Total Prep & Cooking Time: Fifteen minutes
Yields: Four servings
Nutrition Facts: Calories: 722.3 | Protein: 42.3g | Carbs: 0.4g| Fat: 61.5g | Fiber: 0.4g

Ingredients

- Eight lamb chops
- One tbsp. of each
  - Olive oil
  - Butter
- Pepper and salt

For the herb butter:

- Five ounces of butter
- One clove of garlic (mashed)
- Half tbsp. of garlic powder
- Four tbsps. of parsley (chopped)
- One tsp. of lemon juice
- One-third tsp. of salt

Method:

1. Season the lamb chops with pepper and salt.
2. Heat olive oil and butter in an iron skillet. Add the lamb chops. Fry for four minutes.
3. Combine all the listed ingredients for the herb butter in a bowl. Let the herb butter sit for fifteen minutes.
4. Serve the lamb chops with herb butter by the side.

Crispy Cuban Pork Roast

Total Prep & Cooking Time: Nine hours and twenty minutes

Yields: Six servings

Nutrition Facts: Calories: 910.3 | Protein: 58.3g | Carbs: 5.3g| Fat: 69.6g | Fiber: 2.2g

Ingredients

- Five pounds of pork shoulder
- Four tsps. of salt
- Two tsps. of cumin (ground)
- One tsp. of black pepper (ground)
- Two tbsps. of oregano
- One red onion (diced)
- Four cloves of garlic
- One orange (juiced)
- Two lemons (juiced)
- One-fourth cup of olive oil

Method:

1. Rub the pork shoulder with salt. Place the meat in a bowl.
2. Mix all the remaining ingredients of the marinade in a blender.
3. Pour the marinade all over the meat. Marinate in the refrigerator for eight hours.
4. Place the meat in a pressure cooker. Add the marinade.
5. Cook for forty minutes.
6. Preheat your oven at two hundred degrees Celsius.
7. Roast the pork for thirty minutes.
8. Collect the juice from the pressure cooker and boil. Simmer for twenty minutes.
9. Shred the meat using a fork into large chunks.
10. Pour the juice all over the meat.
11. Serve immediately.

Keto Barbecued Ribs

Total Prep & Cooking Time: One hour and forty minutes
Yields: Four servings
Nutrition Facts: Calories: 980.3 | Protein: 54.3g | Carbs: 5.8g| Fat: 80.2g | Fiber: 4.6g

Ingredients

- One-fourth cup of Dijon mustard
- Two tbsps. of each
  - Cider vinegar
  - Butter
  - Salt
- Three pounds of spare ribs
- Four tbsps. of paprika powder
- Half tbsp. of chili powder
- One and a half tbsp. of garlic powder
- Two tsps. of each
  - Onion powder
  - Cumin (ground)
- Two and a half tbsp. of black pepper (ground)

Method:

1. Preheat a grill for thirty minutes.
2. For preparing the wet base, mix vinegar and Dijon mustard in a bowl. Add the ribs and coat well.
3. For preparing the dry rub, mix all the listed spices. Rub the mix all over the ribs. Reserve some for later use.
4. Arrange the coated ribs on an aluminum foil. Add some butter over the ribs.
5. Take the sides of the foil and seal them. Repeat with another foil from outside.
6. Place the wrapped ribs on the preheated grill for one hour. Close the lid.
7. Open the foil and arrange the ribs on a cutting board. Sprinkle reserved spice mix. Return the ribs to the grill. Grill for ten minutes.
8. Serve hot.

Turkey Burgers and Tomato Butter

Total Prep & Cooking Time: Forty minutes Yields: Four servings

Nutrition Facts: Calories: 830.4 | Protein: 33.6g | Carbs: 6.7g| Fat: 71.5g | Fiber: 5.1g

Ingredients

For the chicken patties:

- Two pounds of chicken (ground)
- One large egg
- Half onion (chopped)
- One tsp. of salt
- Half tsp. of black pepper (ground)
- One and a half tsp. of thyme (dried)
- Two ounces of butter

For the fried cabbage:

- Two pounds of green cabbage
- Three ounces of butter
- One tsp. of salt
- Half tsp. of black pepper (ground)

For the tomato butter:

- Four ounces of butter
- One tbsp. of tomato paste
- One tsp. of red wine vinegar
- Pepper and salt

Method:

1. Preheat your oven at one hundred degrees Celsius.
2. Combine the listed ingredients for the patties in a large bowl.
3. Shape the mixture into patties using your hands.
4. Heat butter in an iron skillet. Fry the chicken patties for five minutes on each side.
5. Place the patties in the oven for keeping them warm.
6. Heat butter in a pan. Add the cabbage. Add pepper and salt. Fry for five minutes.
7. Whip the ingredients for the tomato butter in a bowl. Use an electric mixer for even mixing.
8. Arrange the turkey patties on a serving plate. Top with fried cabbage. Serve with a dollop of tomato butter from the top.

Conclusion

I want to thank you for reaching the end of *Keto Diet After 50* . I hope it was full of useful information and capable of providing you all the tools you will require to achieve all the goals.

Now, all you have to do is start with the keto meal plan from the coming week. The quicker you start with the diet plan, the faster you can see the results. Do not just sit and try to figure out the perfect day for starting with the diet. This way, you can never start with the diet plan. If you are waiting for the perfect day, then it is today. As soon as you start with twenty-one days keto meal plan, try your best not to deflect. It is not that tough. Cutting out carbs suddenly might seem to be a bit tough at the beginning. However, once you see the diet plan results after three weeks, you will be amazed. There is nothing too complex about the ketogenic diet. Life after the age of 50 is not at all easy. It will be better for you if you start aiding all the problems from the very beginning.

Just take your grocery bag and go out shopping for all the items that you will need. You can create a shopping list according to the diet meal plan for each week. It will make your task a lot easier. The keto diet has shown positive results after the age of fifties. The recipes that I have included in this book, apart from the keto meal plan recipes, are very easy. You can gather the ingredients from your local grocery store. So, what are you waiting for? Start preparing healthy meals and lead a healthy life after your fifties.

CPSIA information can be obtained
at www.ICGtesting.com
Printed in the USA
LVHW011303010621
689027LV00007B/668

9 780877 679479